Plant Based Cool
Your Lunch & Dinner

Don't Miss These Quick and Easy Recipes to
Make Incredible Plant Based Appetizers

Tanya Lang

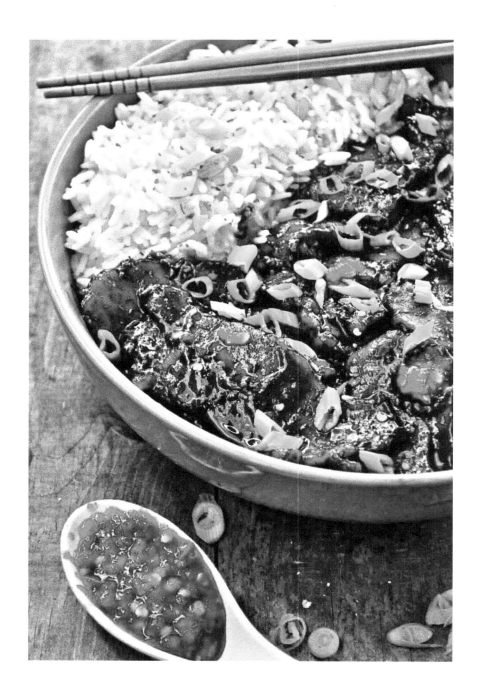

TABLE OF CONTENT

Potato And Pea Stir-Fry 8

Mongolian Seitan 10

Alfredo Pasta With Cherry Tomatoes 12

Tempeh Tetrazzini With Garden Peas 14

Tomato, Kale, and White Bean Skillet 17

Chard Wraps With Millet 19

Quinoa Meatballs 20

Rice Stuffed Jalapeños 22

Pineapple Fried Rice 24

Portobello Kale Florentine 26

Tempeh Oat Balls With Maple Asparagus 28

Chili Mushroom Spaghetti With Watercress 30

Zucchini Rolls In Tomato Sauce 32

Cannellini Beans Bow Ties 34

Crispy Tofu Burgers 36

Green Bean And Mushroom Biryani 38

Cabbage & Bell Pepper Skillet 40

Mixed Bean Burgers With Cashew Cheese 43

Cheesy Bean & Rice Burritos 45

Avocado and Cauliflower Hummus 47

Raw Zoodles with Avocado and Nuts 50

Cauliflower Sushi.. *52*

Pinwheel Greens... *55*

Guacamole Rice and Bean Burritos *57*

Ricotta Basil Pinwheels.. *59*

Delicious Sloppy Joes With No Meat....................... *61*

Coconut Curry Lentils... *63*

Cauliflower-Onion Patties.. *65*

Roasted Garlic Broccoli.. *67*

Carrot Casserole *69*

Carrot-Pineapple Casserole *71*

Broccoli with Garlic Butter and Almonds................ *73*

Roasted Vegetables.. *75*

Honey Roasted Cauliflower *77*

Broccoli Steaks *78*

Roasted Garlic Lemon Cauliflower *81*

Broccoli with Garlic Sauce.. *83*

Cranberry Cabbage... *86*

Deviled Green Beans *88*

Lemon Green Beans with Almonds........................... *90*

Eggplant Casserole *92*

Garlic Green Beans *94*

Ginger Veggie Stir-Fry *96*

Roasted Green Beans *98*

French Fries Made with Zucchini............................ *100*

Garlicky Ginger Eggplant.. *102*

Garlic Kale Buckwheat.. *104*

Glazed Zucchini *106*

Grilled Summer Squash *108*

Pineapple and Pepper Curry *110*

Potato And Pea Stir-Fry

- Preparation Time: 15-30 minutes | Cooking Time: 21 minutes | Servings: 4

Ingredients:

- 4 medium potatoes, peeled and diced
- 2 tbsp olive oil
- 1 medium onion, chopped
- 1 tsp red chili powder
- 1 tsp fresh ginger-garlic paste
- 1 tsp cumin powder
- ¼ tsp turmeric powder
- Salt and black pepper to taste
- 1 cup fresh green peas

Directions:

- Steam potatoes in a safe microwave bowl for 8-10 minutes or until softened. Heat the olive oil in a wok and sauté the onion until softened, 3 minutes.

- Mix in the chili powder, ginger-garlic paste, cumin powder, turmeric powder, salt, and black pepper. Cook until the fragrant releases, 1 minute. Stir in the green peas, potatoes, and cook until softened, 2 to 3 minutes. Serve warm.

Nutrition:

- Calories 394 kcal Fats 7. 7g Carbs 73. 9g Protein 10. 2g

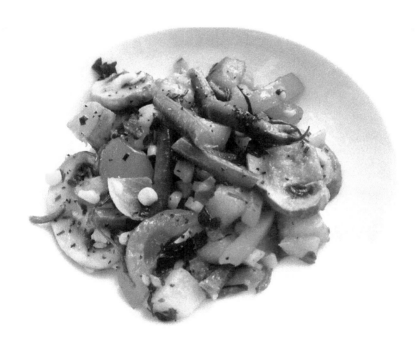

Mongolian Seitan

- Preparation Time: 15-30 minutes | Cooking Time: 20 minutes | Servings: 4

Ingredients:
- For the sauce:
- 2 tsp olive oil
- ½ tsp freshly grated ginger
- 3 garlic cloves, minced
- 1/3 tsp red chili flakes
- 1/3 tsp allspice
- 1/2 cup low-sodium soy sauce
- ½ cup + 2 tbsp pure date sugar
- 2 tsp cornstarch
- 2 tbsp cold water
- For the crisped seitan:
- 1 ½ tbsp olive oil
- 1 lb seitan, cut into 1-inch pieces
- For topping:
- 1 tbsp toasted sesame seeds
- 1 tbsp sliced scallions

Directions:
- Heat the olive oil in a wok and sauté the

ginger and garlic until fragrant, 30 seconds.

• Mix in the red chili flakes, Chinese allspice, soy sauce, and date sugar. Allow the sugar to

melt and set aside.

• In a small bowl, mix the cornstarch and water. Stir the cornstarch mixture into the sauce and allow thickening for 1 minute. Turn the heat off.

• Heat the olive oil in a medium skillet over medium heat and fry the seitan on both sides until crispy, 10 minutes,

• Mix the seitan into the sauce and warm over low heat. Dish the food, garnish with the sesame seeds and scallions. Serve warm with brown rice.

Nutrition:

• Calories 354 kcal Fats 20. 8g Carbs 17. 7g Protein 25. 2g

Alfredo Pasta With Cherry Tomatoes

- Preparation Time: 15-30 minutes | Cooking Time: 20 minutes | Servings: 4

- 2 cups almond milk
- 1 ½ cups vegetable broth
- 3 tbsp plant butter
- 1 large garlic clove, minced
- 16 oz whole-wheat fettuccine
- ½ cup coconut cream
- ¼ cup halved cherry tomatoes
- ¾ cup grated plant-based Parmesan cheese
- Salt and black pepper to taste
- Chopped fresh parsley to garnish

Directions:

• Bring almond milk, vegetable broth, butter, and garlic to a boil in a large pot, 5 minutes. Mix in the fettuccine and cook until tender, while frequently tossing around 10 minutes.

• Mix in coconut cream, tomatoes, plant Parmesan cheese, salt, and pepper. Cook for 3 minutes or until the cheese melts. Garnish with some parsley and serve warm.

Nutrition:
- Calories 698 kcal Fats 26. 1g Carbs 101. 8g Protein 22. 6g

Tempeh Tetrazzini With Garden Peas

- Preparation Time: 15-30 minutes | Cooking Time: 50 minutes | Servings: 4

Ingredients:

- 16 oz whole-wheat bow-tie pasta
- 2 tbsp olive oil, divided
- 2/3 lb tempeh, cut into 1-inch cubes
- Salt and black pepper to taste
- 1 medium yellow onion, chopped
- ½ cup sliced white mushrooms
- 2 tbsp whole-wheat flour
- ¼ cup white wine
- ¾ cup vegetable stock
- ¼ cup oats milk
- 2 tsp chopped fresh thyme
- ¼ cup chopped cauliflower
- ½ cup grated plant-based Parmesan cheese
- 3 tbsp whole-wheat breadcrumbs

Directions:

- Cook the pasta in 8 cups of slightly salted water for 10 minutes or until al dente. Drain and set aside.
- Preheat the oven to 375 F.
- Heat the 1 tbsp of olive oil in a skillet over medium heat, season the tempeh with salt, pepper, and cook until golden brown all around. Mix in onion, mushrooms, and cook until softened, 5 minutes. Stir in flour and cook for 1 more minute. Mix in wine and add two-thirds of the vegetable stock. Cook for 2 minutes while occasionally stirring and then add milk; continue cooking until the sauce thickens, 4 minutes.
- Season with the thyme, salt, black pepper, and half of the Parmesan cheese. Once the cheese melts, turn the heat off and allow cooling.
- Add the rest of the vegetable stock and cauliflower to a food processor and blend until smooth. Pour the mixture into a bowl, pour in the sauce, and mix in pasta until combined.
- Grease a 2 quarts glass baking dish with cooking spray and spread the mixture in the baking dish. Drizzle the remaining olive oil on top, breadcrumbs, some more thyme, and the remaining cheese. Bake

until the cheese melts and is golden brown on top, 30 minutes. Remove the dish from the oven, allow cooling for 3 minutes, and serve.

Nutrition:

• Calories 799 kcal Fats 57. 7g Carbs 54. 3g Protein 27g

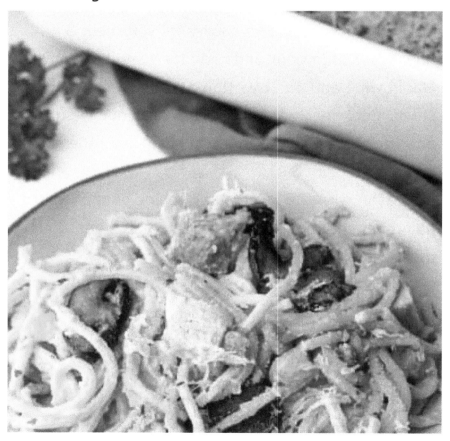

Tomato, Kale, and White Bean Skillet

• Preparation Time: 10 minutes | Cooking Time: 10 minutes | Servings: 4

Ingredients:

- 30 ounces cooked cannellini beans
- 3. 5 ounces sun-dried tomatoes, packed in oil, chopped
- 6 ounces kale, chopped
- 1 teaspoon minced garlic
- 1/4 teaspoon ground black pepper
- 1/4 teaspoon salt
- 1/2 tablespoon dried basil
- 1/8 teaspoon red pepper flakes
- 1 tablespoon apple cider vinegar
- 1 tablespoon olive oil
- 2 tablespoons oil from sun-dried tomatoes

Directions:

• Prepare the dressing and for this, place basil, black pepper, salt, vinegar, and red pepper flakes in a small bowl, add oil from sun-dried tomatoes and whisk until combined.

• Take a skillet pan, place it over medium heat, add olive oil and when hot, add garlic and cook for 1 minute until fragrant.

• Add kale, splash with some water and cook for 3 minutes until kale leaves have wilted.

• Add tomatoes and beans, stir well and cook for 3 minutes until heated.

• Remove pan from heat, drizzle with the prepared dressing, toss until mixed and serve.

Nutrition:

• Calories: 264 Cal Fat: 12 g Carbs: 38 g Protein: 9 g Fiber: 13 g

Chard Wraps With Millet

Preparation Time: 25 minutes | Cooking Time: 0 minute | Servings: 4

- 1 carrot, cut into ribbons
- 1/2 cup millet, cooked
- 1/2 of a large cucumber, cut into ribbons
- 1/2 cup chickpeas, cooked
- 1 cup sliced cabbage
- 1/3 cup hummus
- Mint leaves as needed for topping Hemp seeds as needed for topping 1 bunch of Swiss

rainbow chard

Directions:

- Spread hummus on one side of the chard, place some millet, vegetables, and chickpeas on it, sprinkle with some mint leaves and hemp seeds and wrap it like a burrito.
- Serve straight away.

Nutrition:
- Calories: 152 Cal Fat: 4. 5 g Carbs: 25 g Protein: 3. 5 g Fiber: 2. 4 g

Quinoa Meatballs

- Preparation Time: 10 minutes | Cooking Time: 35 minutes | Servings: 4

Ingredients:

- 1 cup quinoa, cooked
- 1 tablespoon flax meal
- 1 cup diced white onion
- 1 ½ teaspoon minced garlic
- 1/2 teaspoon salt
- 1 teaspoon dried oregano
- 1 teaspoon lemon zest
- 1 teaspoon paprika
- 1 teaspoon dried basil
- 3 tablespoons water
- 2 tablespoons olive oil
- 1 cup grated vegan mozzarella cheese

Marinara sauce as needed for serving
Directions:

- Place flax meal in a bowl, stir in water, and set aside until required.
- Take a large skillet pan, place it over

medium heat, add 1 tablespoon oil and when hot, add

onion and cook for 2 minutes.
• Stir in all the spices and herbs, then stir in quinoa until combined and cook for 2 minutes. • Transfer quinoa mixture in a bowl, add flax meal mixture, lemon zest, and cheese, stir until

well mixed and then shape the mixture into twelve 1 ½ inch balls.
• Arrange balls on a baking sheet lined with parchment paper, refrigerate the balls for 30 minutes and then bake for 20 minutes at 400 degrees F.
• Serve balls with marinara sauce.

Nutrition:
• Calories: 100 Cal Fat: 100 g Carbs: 100 g Protein: 100 g Fiber: 100 g

Rice Stuffed Jalapeños

Preparation Time: 5 minutes | Cooking Time: 15 minutes | Servings: 6

Ingredients:

- 3 medium-sized potatoes, peeled, cubed, boiled
- 2 large carrots, peeled, chopped, boiled
- 3 tablespoons water
- 1/4 teaspoon onion powder
- 1 teaspoons salt
- 1/2 cup nutritional yeast
- 1/4 teaspoon garlic powder
- 1 lime, juiced
- 3 tablespoons water
- Cooked rice as needed
- 3 jalapeños pepper, halved
- 1 red bell pepper, sliced, for garnish
- ½ cup vegetable broth

Directions:

- Place boiled vegetables in a food processor, pour in the broth, and pulse until smooth. • Add garlic powder, onion powder, salt, water, and lime juice, pulse until combined, then add

yeast and blend until smooth.
- Tip the mixture in a bowl, add rice, and stir until incorporated.
- Cut each jalapeno into half lengthwise, brush them with oil, season them with some salt, stuff

them with rice mixture and bake them for 20 minutes at 400 degrees F until done. • Serve straight away.

Nutrition:
- Calories: 148 Cal Fat: 3. 7 g Carbs: 12. 2 g Protein: 2 g Fiber: 2 g

Pineapple Fried Rice

Preparation Time: 5 minutes | Cooking Time: 12 minutes | Servings: 2

Ingredients:

- 2 cups brown rice, cooked
- 1/2 cup sunflower seeds, toasted
- 2/3 cup green peas
- 1 teaspoon minced garlic
- 1 large red bell pepper, cored, diced
- 1 tablespoon grated ginger
- 2/3 cup pineapple chunks with juice
- 2 tablespoons coconut oil
- 1 bunch of green onions, sliced
- For the Sauce:
- 4 tablespoons soy sauce
- 1/2 cup pineapple juice
- 1/2 teaspoon sesame oil
- 1/2 a lime, juiced

Directions:

- Take a skillet pan, place it over medium-high heat, add oil, and when hot, add red bell pepper, pineapple pieces, and two-third of onion, cook for 5 minutes, then stir in ginger and garlic and cook for 1 minute.

- Switch heat to the high level, add rice to the pan, stir until combined, and cook for 5 minutes.
- When done, fold in sunflower seeds and peas and set aside until required.
- Prepare the sauce and for this, place sesame oil in a small bowl, add soy sauce and pineapple juice and whisk until combined.
- Drizzle sauce over rice, drizzle with lime juice and serve straight away.

Nutrition:

- Calories: 179 Cal Fat: 5. 5 g Carbs: 30 g Protein: 3. 3 g Fiber: 2 g

Portobello Kale Florentine

• Preparation Time: 15-30 minutes | Cooking Time: 25 minutes | Servings: 4

Ingredients:

• 4 large portobello mushrooms, stems removed
• 1/8 tsp black pepper
• 1/8 tsp garlic salt
• ½ tsp olive oil
• 1 small onion, chopped
• 1 cup chopped fresh kale
• ¼ cup crumbled tofu cheese
• 1 tbsp chopped fresh basil

Directions:

• Preheat the oven to 350 F and grease a baking sheet with cooking spray.
• Lightly oil the mushrooms with some cooking spray and season with the black pepper and

garlic salt. Arrange the mushrooms on the baking sheet and bake in the oven until tender, 10 to 15 minutes.

• Heat the olive oil in a medium skillet over medium heat and sauté the onion until tender, 3 minutes. Stir in the kale until wilted, 3 minutes. Turn the heat off. Spoon the mixture into the mushrooms and top with the tofu cheese and basil. Serve.

Nutrition:

• Calories 65 kcal Fats 1. 6g Carbs 10. 1g Protein 4. 9g

Tempeh Oat Balls With Maple Asparagus

- Preparation Time: 15-30 minutes | Cooking Time: 40 minutes | Servings: 4 Ingredients:

  - For tempeh balls:
  - 1 tbsp flax seed powder + 3 tbsp water
  - 1 lb tempeh, crumbled
  - ¼ cup chopped red bell pepper
  - Salt and black pepper to taste
  - 1 tbsp almond flour
  - 1 tsp garlic powder
  - 1 tsp onion powder
  - 1 tsp tofu mayonnaise
  - Olive oil for brushing
  - For maple asparagus:
  - 2 tbsp plant butter
  - 1 lb asparagus, hard part trimmed
  - 2 tbsp pure maple syrup
  - 1 tbsp freshly squeezed lemon juice

Directions:
- Preheat the oven to 400 F and line a baking sheet

with parchment paper.

• In a medium bowl, mix the flax seed powder with water and allow thickening for 5 minutes.

Add the tempeh, bell pepper, salt, black pepper, almond flour, garlic powder, onion powder, and tofu mayonnaise. Mix well and form 1-inch balls from the mixture.

• Arrange on the baking sheet, brush with cooking spray, and bake in the oven for 15 to 20 minutes or until brown and compacted. Remove from the oven and set aside for serving.

• Melt the butter in a large skillet and sauté the asparagus until softened with some crunch, 7 minutes. Mix in the maple syrup and lemon juice. Cook for 2 minutes and plate the asparagus. Serve warm with the tempeh balls.

Nutrition:
• Calories 365 kcal Fats 22. 1g Carbs 24. 5g Protein 24. 2g

Chili Mushroom Spaghetti With Watercress

• Preparation Time: 15-30 minutes | Cooking Time: 30 minutes | Servings: 4

Ingredients:

- 1 lb whole-wheat spaghetti
- 3 tbsp plant butter
- 2 tbsp olive oil
- 2 shallots, finely chopped
- 2 garlic cloves, minced
- ½ lb chopped white button mushrooms
- 1 tbsp sake
- 3 tbsp soy sauce
- 1 tsp hot sauce
- A handful of fresh watercress
- ¼ cup chopped fresh parsley
- Black pepper to taste

Directions:

• Cook the spaghetti in slightly salted water in a large pot over medium heat until al dente, 10 minutes. Drain the spaghetti and set aside.

• Heat the butter and olive oil in a large skillet over medium heat and sauté the shallots, garlic, and mushrooms until softened, 5 minutes.

• Stir in the sake, soy sauce, and hot sauce. Cook further for 1 minute.

• Toss the spaghetti in the sauce along with the watercress and parsley. Cook for 1 minute and season with the black pepper. Dish the food and serve warm.

Nutrition:

• Calories 393 kcal Fats 22. 2g Carbs 42. 9g Protein 9. 3g

Zucchini Rolls In Tomato Sauce

• Preparation Time: 15-30 minutes | Cooking Time: 60 minutes | Servings: 4

Ingredients:

- 3 large zucchinis, sliced lengthwise into strips
- Salt and black pepper to taste
- 1 tbsp olive oil
- ¾ lb crumbled tempeh
- 1 cup crumbled tofu cheese
- 1/3 cup grated plant-based Parmesan cheese
- ¼ cup chopped fresh basil leaves
- 2 garlic cloves, minced
- 1 ½ cups marinara sauce, divided
- 2 cups shredded plant-based mozzarella, divided

Directions:

• Line a baking sheet with paper towels and lay the zucchini slices in a single layer on the sheet. Sprinkle each side with some salt and allow the release of liquid for 15 minutes.

• Heat the olive oil in a large skillet over medium

heat and cook the tempeh until browned, 10 minutes. Set aside.

• In a medium bowl, mix the tempeh, tofu cheese, plant Parmesan cheese, basil, and garlic; season with salt and black pepper.

• Preheat the oven to 400 F.

• Spread 1 cup of marinara sauce onto the bottom of a 10-inch oven-proof skillet and set aside.

• Spread 1 tbsp of the cheese mixture evenly along with each zucchini slice; sprinkle with 1 tbsp of plant mozzarella cheese. Roll up the zucchini slices over the filling and arrange them in the skillet. Top with the remaining ½ cup of marinara sauce and sprinkle with the remaining plant mozzarella.

• Bake in the oven for 25-30 minutes or until the zucchini rolls are heated through and the cheese begins to brown. Serve immediately.

Nutrition:
• Calories 428 kcal Fats 14. 5g Carbs 31. 3g Protein 40. 3g

Cannellini Beans Bow Ties

• Preparation Time: 15-30 minutes | Cooking Time: 35 minutes | Servings: 4

Ingredients:

- 2 ½ cups whole-wheat bow tie pasta
- 1 tbsp olive oil
- 1 medium zucchini, sliced
- 2 garlic cloves, minced
- 2 large tomatoes, chopped
- 1 (15 oz) can cannellini beans, rinsed and drained
- 1 (2 ¼ oz) can pitted green olives, sliced
- ½ cup crumbled tofu cheese

Directions:

• Cook the pasta in 8 cups of slightly salted water in a medium pot over medium heat until al dente, 10 minutes. Drain the pasta and set aside.

• Heat olive oil in a skillet and sauté zucchini and garlic for 4 minutes. Stir in tomatoes, beans, and olives. Cook until the tomatoes soften, 10 minutes. Mix in pasta. Allow warming for 1 minute. Stir in tofu cheese and serve warm.

Nutrition:

- Calories 206 kcal Fats 5. 1g Carbs 35. 8g Protein 7. 6g

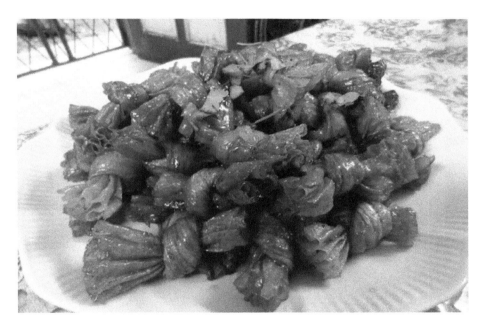

Crispy Tofu Burgers

- Preparation Time: 15-30 minutes | Cooking Time: 20 minutes | Servings: 4

Ingredients:

- 1 tbsp flax seed powder + 3 tbsp water
- 2/3 lb crumble tofu
- 1 tbsp quick-cooking oats
- 1 tbsp toasted almond flour
- ½ tsp garlic powder
- ½ tsp onion powder
- Salt and black pepper to taste
- ¼ tsp curry powder
- 3 tbsp whole-grain breadcrumbs
- 4 whole-wheat burger buns, halved

Directions:

- In a small bowl, mix the flax seed powder with water and allow thickening for 5 minutes to make the flax egg. Set aside.
- In a medium bowl, mix the tofu, oats, almond flour, garlic powder, onion powder, salt, black pepper, and curry powder. Mold 4 patties out of the mixture and lightly brush both sides with the flax

egg.

• Pour the breadcrumbs onto a plate and coat the patties in the crumbs until well covered. • Heat a pan to medium heat and grease well with cooking spray.

• Cook the patties on both sides until crispy, golden brown, and cooked through, 10 minutes. • Place each patty between each burger bun and top with the guacamole.

• Serve immediately.

Nutrition:

• Calories 238 kcal Fats 15. 8g Carbs 14. 8g Protein 14. 1g

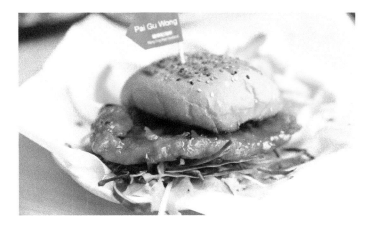

Green Bean And Mushroom Biryani

- Preparation Time: 15-30 minutes | Cooking Time: 50 minutes | Servings: 4

Ingredients:
- 1 cup of brown rice
- 2 cups of water
- Salt to taste
- 3 tbsp plant butter
- 3 medium white onions, chopped
- 6 garlic cloves, minced
- 1 tsp ginger puree
- 1 tbsp turmeric powder + more for dusting
- ¼ tsp cinnamon powder
- 2 tsp garam masala
- ½ tsp cardamom powder
- ½ tsp cayenne powder
- ½ tsp cumin powder
- 1 tsp smoked paprika
- 3 large tomatoes, diced
- 2 green chilies, deseeded and minced

- 1 tbsp tomato puree
- 1 cup chopped cremini mushrooms
- 1 cup chopped mustard greens
- 1 cup plant-based yogurt for topping

Directions:

- Melt the butter in a large pot and sauté the onions until softened, 3 minutes. Mix in the garlic, ginger, turmeric, cardamom powder, garam masala, cardamom powder, cayenne pepper, cumin powder, paprika, and salt. Stir-fry while cooking until fragrant, 1 to 2 minutes.
- Stir in the tomatoes, green chili, tomato puree, and mushrooms. Once boiling, mix in the rice and cover with water. Cover the pot and cook over medium heat until the liquid absorbs and the rice is tender, 15-20 minutes.
- Open the lid and fluff in the mustard greens and half of the parsley. Dish the food, top with the coconut yogurt, garnish with the remaining parsley and serve warm.

Nutrition:

- Calories 255 Fats 16. 8g Carbs 25. 6g Protein 5. 8g

Cabbage & Bell Pepper Skillet

- Preparation Time: 15-30 minutes | Cooking Time: 30 minutes | Servings: 4

Ingredients:
- 1 can (28 oz) whole plum tomatoes, undrained
- 1 lb crumbled tempeh
- 1 large yellow onion, chopped
- 1 can (8 oz) tomato sauce
- 2 tbsp plain vinegar
- 1 tbsp pure date sugar
- 1 tsp dried mixed herbs
- 3 large tomatoes, chopped
- ½ tsp black pepper
- 1 small head cabbage, thinly sliced
- 1 medium green bell pepper, deseeded and cut into thin strips

Directions:
- Drain the tomatoes and reserve their liquid. Chop the tomatoes and set them

aside. • Add the tempeh to a large skillet and cook until brown, 10 minutes. Mix in the onion, tomato

sauce, vinegar, date sugar, mixed herbs, and chopped tomatoes. Close the lid and cook until the liquid reduces and the tomato softens for about 10 minutes.

• Stir in the cabbage and bell pepper; cook until softened, 5 minutes.

- Dish the food and serve it with cooked brown rice.

Nutrition:

- Calories 403 Fats 16. 9g Carbs 44. 1g Protein 27. 3g

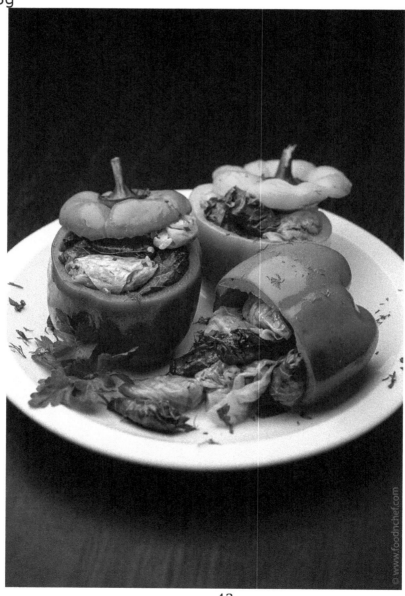

Mixed Bean Burgers With Cashew Cheese

• Preparation Time: 15-30 minutes | Cooking Time: 30 minutes | Servings: 4

Ingredients:

- 1 (15 oz) can chickpea, drained and rinsed
- 1 (15 oz) can pinto beans, drained and rinsed
- 1 (15 oz) can red kidney beans, drained and rinsed
- 2 tbsp whole-wheat flour
- ¼ cup dried mixed herbs
- ¼ tsp hot sauce
- ½ tsp garlic powder
- Salt and black pepper to taste
- 4 slices cashew cheese
- 4 whole-grain hamburger buns, split
- 4 small lettuce leaves for topping
- In a medium bowl, mash the chickpea, pinto beans, kidney beans and mix in the flour, mixed

herbs, hot sauce, garlic powder, salt, and black pepper. Mold 4 patties out of the mixture and set aside.

• Heat a grill pan to medium heat and lightly grease with cooking spray.

• Cook the bean patties on both sides until light brown and cooked through, 10 minutes.

• Lay a cashew cheese slice on each and allow slight melting, 2 minutes.

• Remove the patties between the burger buns and top with the lettuce and serve warm.

Nutrition:

• Calories 456 Fats 16. 8g Carbs 56. 1g Protein 24g

Cheesy Bean & Rice Burritos

• Preparation Time: 15-30 minutes | Cooking Time: 50 minutes | Servings: 4

Ingredients:

- 1 cups brown rice
- Salt and black pepper to taste
- 1 tbsp olive oil
- 1 medium red onion, chopped
- 1 medium green bell pepper, deseeded and diced
- 2 garlic cloves, minced
- 1 tbsp chili powder
- 1 tsp cumin powder
- 1/8 tsp red chili flakes
- 1 (15 oz) can black beans, rinsed and drained
- 4 (8-inch) whole-wheat flour tortillas, warmed
- 1 cup of salsa
- 1 cup coconut cream for topping
- 1 cup grated plant-based cheddar cheese for topping

Directions:

- Add 2 cups of water and brown rice to a medium pot, season with some salt, and cook over medium heat until the water absorbs and the rice is tender, 15 to 20 minutes.
- Heat the olive oil in a medium skillet over medium heat and sauté the onion, bell pepper, and garlic until softened and fragrant, 3 minutes.
- Mix in the chili powder, cumin powder, red chili flakes, and season with salt and black pepper. Cook for 1 minute or until the food releases fragrance. Stir in the brown rice, black beans, and allow warming through, 3 minutes.
- Lay the tortillas on a clean, flat surface and divide the rice mixture in the center of each. Top with the salsa, coconut cream, and plant cheddar cheese. Fold the sides and ends of the tortillas over the filling to secure. Serve immediately.

Nutrition:
- Calories 421 Fats 29. 1g Carbs 37g Protein 9. 3g

Avocado and Cauliflower Hummus

Preparation Time: 5 minutes | Cooking Time: 25 minutes | Servings: 2

Ingredients:

- 1 medium cauliflower, stem removed and chopped
- 1 large Hass avocado, peeled, pitted, and chopped
- ¼ cup extra virgin olive oil
- 2 garlic cloves
- ½ tbsp. lemon juice
- ½ tsp. onion powder
- Sea salt and ground black pepper to taste
- 2 large carrots
- ¼ cup fresh cilantro, chopped

Directions:

- Preheat the oven to 450°F, and line a baking tray with aluminum foil.
- Put the chopped cauliflower on the

baking tray and drizzle with 2 tablespoons of olive oil. • Roast the chopped cauliflower in the oven for 20-25 minutes, until lightly brown. • Remove the tray from the oven and allow the cauliflower to cool down.

• Add all the ingredients—except the carrots and optional fresh cilantro—to a food processor

or blender, and blend the ingredients into a smooth hummus.

• Transfer the hummus to a medium-sized bowl, cover, and put it in the fridge for at least 30 minutes.

• Take the hummus out of the fridge and, if desired, top it with the optional chopped cilantro and more salt and pepper to taste; serve with the carrot fries, and enjoy!

Nutrition:

• Calories 416 Carbohydrates 8. 4 g Fats 40. 3 g Protein 3. 3 g

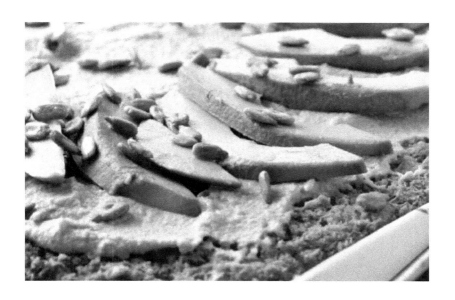

Raw Zoodles with Avocado and Nuts

• Preparation Time: 10 minutes | Cooking Time: 3-30 minutes | Servings: 2

Ingredients:
- 1 medium zucchini
- 1½ cups basil
- 1/3 cup water
- 5 tbsp. pine nuts
- 2 tbsp. lemon juice
- 1 medium avocado, peeled, pitted, sliced
- Optional: 2 tbsp. olive oil
- 6 yellow cherry tomatoes, halved
- Optional: 6 red cherry tomatoes, halved
- Sea salt and black pepper to taste
- Add the basil, water, nuts, lemon juice, avocado slices, optional olive oil (if desired), salt,

and pepper to a blender.

• Blend the ingredients into a smooth mixture. Add more salt and pepper to taste and blend again.

• Divide the sauce and the zucchini noodles between two medium-sized bowls for serving, and combine in each.

• Top the mixtures with the halved yellow cherry tomatoes, and the optional red cherry tomatoes (if desired); serve and enjoy!

Nutrition:

• Calories 317 Carbohydrates 7. 4 g Fats 28. 1 g Protein 7. 2 g

Cauliflower Sushi

- Preparation Time: 30 minutes | Cooking Time: 3-30 minutes | Servings: 4

Ingredients:

- Sushi Base:
- 6 cups cauliflower florets
- ½ cup vegan cheese
- 1 medium spring onion, diced
- 4 nori sheets
- Sea salt and pepper to taste
- 1 tbsp. rice vinegar or sushi vinegar
- 1 medium garlic clove, minced
- Filling:
- 1 medium Hass avocado, peeled, sliced
- ½ medium cucumber, skinned, sliced
- 4 asparagus spears
- A handful of enoki mushrooms

Directions:

- Put the cauliflower florets in a food processor or blender. Pulse the florets into a rice-like substance. When using ready-made cauliflower rice, add this to the blender.

- Add the vegan cheese, spring onions, and vinegar to the food processor or blender. Top these ingredients with salt and pepper to taste, and pulse everything into a chunky mixture. Make sure not to turn the ingredients into a puree by pulsing too long.
- Taste and add more vinegar, salt, or pepper to taste. Add the optional minced garlic clove to the blender and pulse again for a few seconds.
- Lay the nori sheets and spread the cauliflower rice mixture out evenly between the sheets. Make sure to leave at least 2 inches of the top and bottom edges empty.
- Place one or more combinations of multiple filling ingredients along the center of the spreadout rice mixture. Experiment with different ingredients per nori sheet for the best flavor.
- Roll up each nori sheet tightly. (Using a sushi mat will make this easier.)
- Either serve the sushi as a nori roll or, slice each roll up into sushi pieces.
- Serve right away with a small amount of wasabi, pickled ginger, and soy sauce!

Nutrition:

- Calories 189 Carbohydrates 7. 6 g Fats 14. 4 g
Protein 6. 1 g

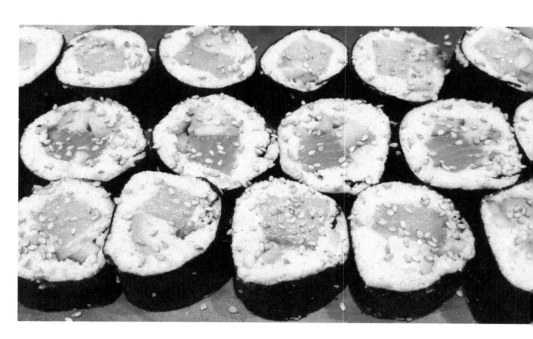

Pinwheel Greens

Preparation Time: 5 minutes | Cooking Time: 1 minute | Servings: 16

Ingredients:

- ½ cup of water
- 4 tablespoons white vinegar
- 3 tablespoons lemon juice
- 3 tablespoons tahini paste
- 1 clove garlic, minced
- Salt and pepper to taste
- Canned artichokes, drained, thinly sliced
- Cherry tomatoes, thinly sliced
- Olives, thinly sliced
- Lettuce or baby spinach
- Tortillas

Directions:

• In a bowl, combine the water, vinegar, lemon juice, and Tahini paste; whisk together until smooth.

• Add the garlic, salt, and pepper to taste; whisk to combine. Set the bowl aside.

• Lay a tortilla on a flat surface and spread with

one tablespoon of the sauce.

• Lay some lettuce or spinach slices on top, then scatter some artichoke, tomato, and olive slices on top.

• Tightly roll the tortilla and fold in the sides. Cut the ends off and then slice into four or five pinwheels.

Nutrition:

• Calories 322 Carbohydrates 5g Fats 4g Protein 30g

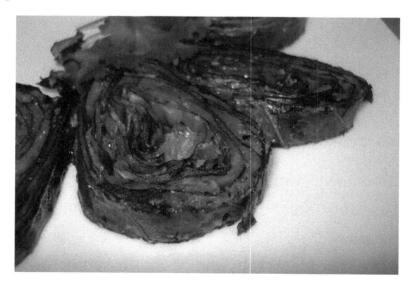

Guacamole Rice and Bean Burritos

• Preparation Time: 10 minutes | Cooking Time: 15 minutes | Servings: 8

Ingredients:
- 2 16-ounce cans fat-free refried beans
- 6 tortillas
- 2 cups cooked rice
- ½ cup of salsa
- 1 tablespoon olive oil
- 1 bunch green onions, chopped
- 2 bell peppers, finely chopped
- Guacamole

Directions:
- Preheat the oven to 375°F.
- Dump the refried beans into a saucepan and place over medium heat to warm. • Heat the tortillas and lay them out on a flat surface.
- Spoon the beans in a long mound that runs across the tortilla, just a little off from

the center. • Spoon some rice and salsa over the beans; add the green pepper and onions to taste, along

with any other finely chopped vegetables you like.
• Fold over the shortest edge of the plain tortilla and roll it up, folding in the sides as you go. • Place each burrito, seam side down, on a baking sheet sprayed with a non-stick spray. • Brush with olive oil and bake for 15 minutes.
• Serve with guacamole.

Nutrition:
• Calories 290 Carbohydrates 49 g Fats 6 g Protein 9 g

Ricotta Basil Pinwheels

- Preparation Time: 10 minutes | Cooking Time: 3-30 minutes | Servings: 4

Ingredients:

- ½ cup unsalted cashews
- Water
- 7 ounces firm tofu, cut into pieces
- ¼ cup almond milk
- 1 teaspoon white wine vinegar
- 1 clove garlic, smashed
- 20 to 25 fresh basil leaves
- Salt and pepper to taste
- 8 tortillas
- 7 ounces fresh spinach
- ½ cup black olives, sliced
- 2 to 3 tomatoes, cut into small pieces

Directions:

• Soak the cashews for 30 minutes in enough water to cover them. Drain them well and pat them dry with paper towels.

• Place the cashews in a blender along with the tofu, almond milk, vinegar, garlic, basil leaves, salt, and pepper to taste. Blend until smooth and creamy.

 • Spread the resulting mixture on the eight tortillas, dividing it equally.

 • Top with spinach leaves, olives, and tomatoes.

 • Tightly roll each loaded tortilla.

 • Cut off the ends with a sharp knife and slice into four or five pinwheels.

Nutrition:

 • Calories 236 Carbohydrates 6. 1 g Fats 21.Protein 4. 2 g

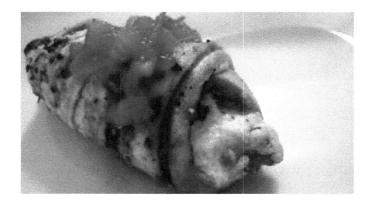

Delicious Sloppy Joes With No Meat

Preparation Time: 6 minutes | Cooking Time: 5 minutes | Servings: 4

Ingredients:

- 5 tablespoons vegetable stock
- 2 stalks celery, diced
- 1 small onion, diced
- 1 small red bell pepper, diced
- 1 teaspoon garlic powder
- 1 teaspoon chili powder
- 1 teaspoon ground cumin
- 1 teaspoon salt
- 1 cup cooked bulgur wheat
- 1 cup red lentils
- 1 15-ounce can tomato sauce
- 4 tablespoons tomato paste
- 3½ cups water
- 2 teaspoons balsamic vinegar
- 1 tablespoon Hoisin sauce

Directions:

• In a Dutch oven, heat the vegetable stock and add the celery, onion, and bell pepper. Sauté until vegetables are soft, about five minutes.

• Add the garlic powder, chili powder, cumin, and salt and mix in.

• Add the bulgur wheat, lentils, tomato sauce, tomato paste, water, vinegar, and Hoisin sauce. Stir and bring to a boil.

• Turn the heat down to a simmer and cook uncovered for 30 minutes. Stir occasionally to prevent sticking and scorching.

• Taste to see if the lentils are tender.

• When the lentils are done, serve on buns.

Nutrition:

• Calories 451 Fats 10 g Carbohydrates 61 g Protein 27 g

Coconut Curry Lentils

- Preparation Time: 10 minutes | Cooking Time: 40 minutes | Servings: 4

Ingredients:
- 1 cup brown lentils
- 1 small white onion, peeled, chopped
- 1 teaspoon minced garlic
- 1 teaspoon grated ginger
- 3 cups baby spinach
- 1 tablespoon curry powder
- 2 tablespoons olive oil
- 13 ounces coconut milk, unsweetened
- 2 cups vegetable broth
- For Servings:

- 4 cups cooked rice
- 1/4 cup chopped cilantro

Directions:
- Place a large pot over medium heat, add oil and when hot, add ginger and garlic and cook for

1 minute until fragrant.
- Add onion, cook for 5 minutes, stir in curry powder, cook for 1 minute until toasted, add

lentils, and pour in broth.

• Switch heat to medium-high level, bring the mixture to a boil, then switch heat to the low level and simmer for 20 minutes until tender and all the liquid is absorbed.

• Pour in milk, stir until combined, turn heat to medium level, and simmer for 10 minutes until thickened.

• Then remove the pot from heat, stir in spinach, let it stand for 5 minutes until its leaves wilts and then top with cilantro.

• Serve lentils with rice.

Nutrition:

• Calories: 184 Cal Fat: 3. 7 g Carbs: 30 g Protein: 11. 3 g Fiber: 10. 7 g

Cauliflower-Onion Patties

• Preparation Time: 05 minutes | Cooking Time: 10 minutes | Servings: 4

Ingredients:
- 3 cups cauliflower florets
- 1/2 cup onion
- 2 large eggs
- 2 tablespoons all-purpose white flour
- 2 tablespoons olive oil

Directions:
- Dice cauliflower and chop onion.
- Boil the diced cauliflower in a small amount of water for 5 minutes; drain.
- Break eggs into a medium bowl and beat. Add the flour and mix well.
- Add the cauliflower and onion and stir into the flour/egg mixture until well mixed.
- Add olive oil to a frying pan and heat.
- Drop the mixture by spoonful's into the hot oil, making 4 equal portions (or 8 portions

smaller size are desired).

• Using a spatula, flatten the latkes and fry until brown on both sides.

• Drain on a paper towel to soak up extra oil.

• Serve hot.

Nutrition:

• Calories 134, Total Fat 9.6g, Saturated Fat 1.8g, Cholesterol 93mg, Sodium 58mg, Total Carbohydrate 8.5g, Dietary Fiber 2.3g, Total Sugars 2.6g, Protein 5.2g, Calcium 34mg, Iron 1mg, Potassium 286mg, Phosphorus 229 mg

Roasted Garlic Broccoli

• Preparation Time: 15 minutes | Cooking Time: 25 minutes | Servings: 4

Ingredients:
- 2 tablespoons minced garlic
- 3 tablespoons olive oil
- 1 large head broccoli, separated into florets
- 1/3 cup grated Parmesan cheese
- Salt and black pepper to taste
- 1 tablespoon chopped fresh basil

Directions:

• Preheat the oven to 450 degrees F. Grease a large casserole dish.

• Place the olive oil and garlic in a large resealable bag. Add broccoli, and shake to mix. Pour

into the prepared casserole dish, and season with salt and pepper to taste.

• Bake for 25 minutes, stirring halfway through. Top with Parmesan cheese and

basil, and broil

for 3 to 5 minutes, until golden brown.

Nutrition:

• Calories 112, Total Fat 11.1g, Saturated Fat 1.8g, Cholesterol 2mg, Sodium 30mg, Total Carbohydrate 3g, Dietary Fiber 0.7g, Total Sugars 0.4g, Protein 1.7g, Calcium 40mg, Iron 0mg, Potassium 91mg Phosphorus 89 mg

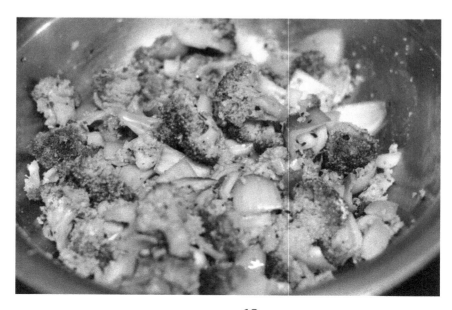

Carrot Casserole

- Preparation Time: 15 minutes | Cooking Time: 15 minutes | Servings: 4

Ingredients:
- ½ pound carrots
- ½ cup graham crackers
- 1 tablespoon olive oil
- 1 tablespoon onion
- 1/8 teaspoon black pepper
- 1/6 cup shredded cheddar cheese
- Salt

Directions:
- Preheat the oven to 350º F.
- Peel carrots and slice into 1/4-inch rounds. Place carrots in a large saucepan over mediumhigh heat and boil until soft enough to mash. Drain and reserve 1/3-cup liquid.

- Mash carrots until they are smooth.

- Crush graham crackers, heat oil, and minced onion. Stir crackers, onion, oil, salt, pepper, and reserved liquid into mashed carrots.

• Place in a greased small casserole dish. Sprinkle shredded cheese on top and bake for 15 minutes. Serve hot.

Nutrition:

• Calories 118, Total Fat 6.1g, Saturated Fat 1.7g, Cholesterol 5mg, Sodium 86mg, Total Carbohydrate 14g, Dietary Fiber 1.8g, Total Sugars 6.2g, Protein 2.4g, Calcium 56mg, Iron 1mg, Potassium 205mg, Phosphorus 189 mg

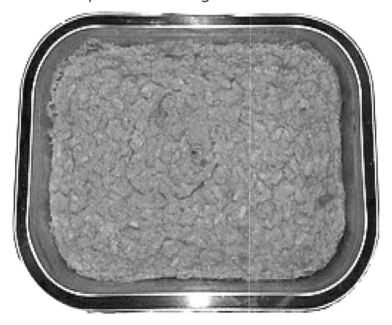

Carrot-Pineapple Casserole

• Preparation Time: 10 minutes | Cooking Time: 50 minutes | Servings: 4

Ingredients:
- 3 large carrots
- 1 large pineapple
- 2 tablespoons all-purpose flour
- 1 tablespoon honey
- ½ teaspoon ground cinnamon
- 1 tablespoon olive oil
- 1/2 cup pineapple juice

Directions:
- Preheat the oven to 350 degrees F.
- Peel and slice carrots and pineapples.

Bring 1 quart of water to a boil in a medium-sized pot.

Boil carrots for 5 minutes or until tender. Drain.
- Layer carrots and pineapples in a large casserole dish.
- Using a fork, mix flour, honey, and

cinnamon in a small bowl. Mix in olive oil to make a

crumb topping.

• Sprinkle flour mixture over carrots and pineapples then drizzle with juice.

• Bake for 50 minutes or until pineapples and carrots are tender and the topping is golden

brown.

Nutrition:

• Calories 94, Total Fat 2.9g, Saturated Fat 0.4g, Cholesterol 0mg, Sodium 31mg, Total Carbohydrate 17.4g, Dietary Fiber 1.8g, Total Sugars 11.2g, Protein 0.9g, Calcium 23mg, Iron 0mg, Potassium 206mg, Phosphorus 27 mg

Broccoli with Garlic Butter and Almonds

• Preparation Time: 10 minutes | Cooking Time: 50 minutes | Servings: 4

Ingredients:

- 1 pound fresh broccoli, cut into bite-size pieces
- ¼ cup olive oil
- ½ tablespoon honey
- 1-1/2 tablespoons soy sauce
- ¼ teaspoon ground black pepper
- 2 cloves garlic, minced
- ¼ cup chopped almonds

Directions:

• Place the broccoli into a large pot with about 1 inch of water in the bottom. Bring to a boil, and cook for 7 minutes, or until tender but still crisp. Drain, and arrange broccoli on a serving platter.

• While the broccoli is cooking, heat the oil in a small skillet over medium heat. Mix in the honey, soy sauce, pepper, and garlic. Bring to a boil, then remove from the heat. Mix in the almonds, and pour the sauce over the broccoli. Serve immediately.

Nutrition:
• Calories 177, Total Fat 17.3g, Saturated Fat 2.1g, Cholesterol 0mg, Sodium 234mg, Total Carbohydrate 5.3g, Dietary Fiber 1.2g, Total Sugars 2.7g, Protein 2.9g, Calcium 20mg, Iron 1mg, Potassium 131mg, Phosphorus 67 mg

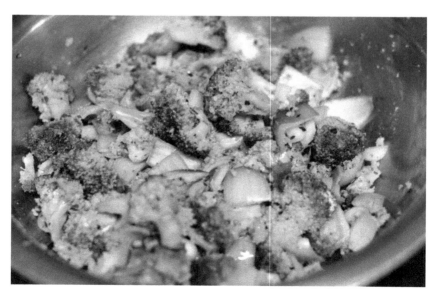

Roasted Vegetables

• Preparation Time: 15 minutes | Cooking Time: 40 minutes | Servings: 4

Ingredients:

- ¼ summer squash, cubed
- 1 red bell peppers, seeded and diced
- 1 red onion, quartered
- ¼ cup green beans
- 1 tablespoon chopped fresh thyme
- 2 tablespoons chopped fresh rosemary
- 1/4 cup olive oil
- ½ tablespoon lemon juice
- Salt and freshly ground black pepper

Directions:

- Preheat the oven to 475 degrees F.
- In a large bowl, combine the squash, red bell peppers, and green beans. Separate the red

onion quarters into pieces, and add them to the mixture.

- In a small bowl, stir together thyme,

rosemary, olive oil, lemon juice, salt, and pepper. Toss
 with vegetables until they are coated. Spread evenly on a large roasting pan. • Roast for 35 to 40 minutes in the preheated oven, stirring every 10 minutes, or until
 vegetables are cooked through and browned.

Nutrition:
• Calories 145, Total Fat 13.1g, Saturated Fat 2g, Cholesterol 0mg, Sodium 4mg, Total Carbohydrate 8g, Dietary Fiber 2.5g, Total Sugars 3.5g, Protein 1.3g, Calcium 47mg, Iron 2mg, Potassium 160mg, Phosphorus 110mg

Honey Roasted Cauliflower

- Preparation Time: 10 minutes | Cooking Time: 35 minutes | Servings: 4

Ingredients:

- 2 cups cauliflower
- 2 tablespoons diced onion
- 2 tablespoons olive oil
- 1 tablespoon honey
- 1 teaspoon dry mustard
- 1 pinch salt
- 1 pinch ground black pepper

Directions:

- Preheat the oven to 375 degrees F. Lightly coat an 11x7 inch baking dish with non-stick cooking spray.
- Place cauliflower in a single layer in a prepared dish, and top with onion. In a small bowl, combine olive oil, honey, mustard, salt, and pepper; drizzle over cauliflower and onion.
- Bake in the preheated 375 degrees F

oven for 35 minutes or until tender, stirring halfway through the cooking time.

Nutrition:

- Calories 88, Total Fat 7.3g, Saturated Fat 1g, Cholesterol 0mg, Sodium 47mg, Total Carbohydrate 6.4g, Dietary Fiber 0.9g, Total Sugars 5.2g, Protein 0.8g, Calcium 11mg, Iron 0mg, Potassium 92mg, Phosphorus 70mg

Broccoli Steaks

- Preparation Time: 10 minutes | Cooking Time: 25 minutes | Servings: 4

Ingredients:

- 1 medium head broccoli
- 3 tablespoons unsalted butter
- ¼ teaspoon garlic powder
- ¼ teaspoon onion powder
- 1/8 teaspoon salt
- ¼ teaspoon pepper

Directions:

- Preheat the oven to 400 degrees F.

Please parchment paper on a roasting pan.

• Trim the leaves off the broccoli and cut off the bottom of the stem. Cut the broccoli head in

half. Cut each half into 1 to 3/4-inch slices, leaving the core in place. Cut off the smaller ends of the broccoli and save for another recipe. There should be 4 broccoli steaks. • Mix butter, garlic powder, onion powder, salt, and pepper.

• Lay the broccoli on the parchment-lined baking sheet. Using half of the butter mixture, brush onto the steaks. Place in the preheated oven for 20 minutes. Remove from the oven and flip the steaks over. Brush steaks with remaining butter and roast for about 20 more minutes, until they are golden brown on the edges.

Nutrition:

• Calories 86, Total Fat 8.7g, Saturated Fat 5.5g, Cholesterol 23mg, Sodium 143mg, Total Carbohydrate 1.9g, Dietary Fiber 0.7g, Total Sugars 0.5g, Protein 0.8g,

Calcium 15mg, Iron 0mg, Potassium 80mg, Phosphorus 61 mg

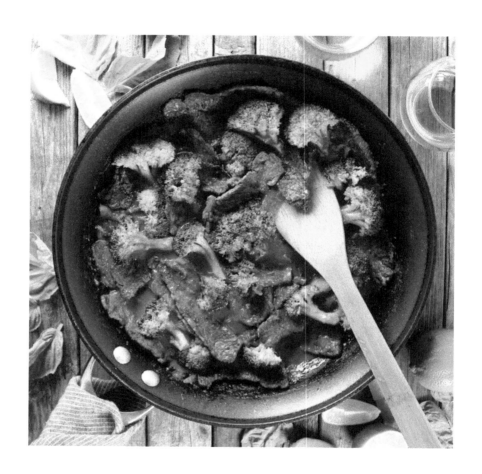

Roasted Garlic Lemon Cauliflower

• Preparation Time: 10 minutes | Cooking Time: 15 minutes | Servings: 4

Ingredients:

• 2 heads cauliflower, separated into florets

• 2 teaspoons olive oil

• ½ teaspoon ground black pepper

• 1 clove garlic, minced

• ½ teaspoon lemon juice

Directions:

• Preheat the oven to 400 degrees F.

• In a large bowl, toss broccoli florets with olive oil, pepper, and garlic. Spread the broccoli out

in an even layer on a baking sheet.

• Bake in the preheated oven until florets are tender enough to pierce the stems with a fork, 15

to 20 minutes. Remove and transfer to a

serving platter. Squeeze lemon juice liberally over
 the broccoli before serving for a refreshing, tangy finish.

Nutrition:

• Calories 37, Total Fat 1.7g, Saturated Fat 0.2g, Cholesterol 0mg, Sodium 27mg, Total Carbohydrate 5g, Dietary Fiber 2.3g, Total Sugars 2.1g, Protein 1.8g, Calcium 21mg, Iron 0mg, Potassium 272mg, Phosphorus 161 mg

Broccoli with Garlic Sauce

• Preparation Time: 10 minutes | Cooking Time: 15 minutes | Servings: 4

Ingredients:
- 2 cups broccoli florets
- 1 garlic cloves
- ½ tablespoon butter
- 2 teaspoons honey
- 1-1/2 tablespoons apple cider vinegar
- 1 tablespoon fresh parsley

Directions:

• In a large saucepan with a steamer rack, steam broccoli over boiling water for 8 to 10 minutes or until crisp-tender (cover with a lid while steaming).

• In a small saucepan, cook minced garlic in butter for 30 seconds then remove the pan from heat.

• Stir in honey, apple cider vinegar, and chopped parsley. Return the saucepan to heat until the sauce is heated.

• Transfer steamed broccoli to a serving dish.

• Pour sauce over hot broccoli and toss to coat.

Nutrition:

• Calories 41, Total Fat 1.6g, Saturated Fat 0.9g, Cholesterol 4mg, Sodium 26mg, Total Carbohydrate 6.2g, Dietary Fiber 1.2g, Total Sugars 3.7g, Protein 1.4g, Calcium 25mg, Iron 0mg, Potassium 157mg, Phosphorus 100 mg

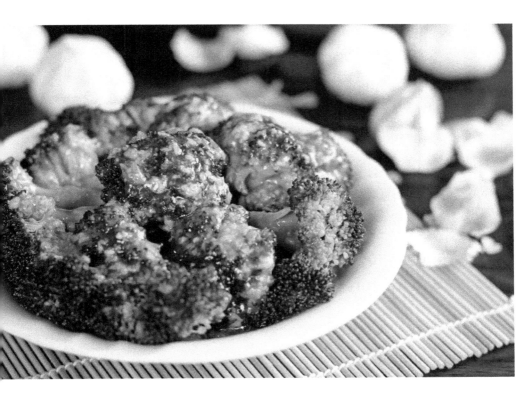

Cranberry Cabbage

- Preparation Time: 10 minutes | Cooking Time: 15 minutes | Servings: 4

Ingredients:

- 8 ounces canned whole-berry cranberry sauce
- 1 tablespoon fresh lemon juice
- 1/4 teaspoon ground cloves
- 1 medium head red cabbage

Directions:

- In a large pan heat cranberry sauce, lemon juice, and cloves together and bring to a simmer. • Stir cabbage into melted cranberry sauce, mixing well. Bring mixture to a boil; reduce heat to

simmer. Continue cooking until cabbage is tender, stirring occasionally.
- Serve hot.

Nutrition:

- Calories 38, Total Fat 0.1g, Saturated Fat 0g, Cholesterol 0mg, Sodium 20mg, Total Carbohydrate 7.9g, Dietary Fiber 2.6g,

Total Sugars 3.8g, Protein 1g, Calcium 37mg, Iron 1mg, Potassium 224mg, Phosphorus 120 mg

Deviled Green Beans

- Preparation Time: 10 minutes | Cooking Time: 15 minutes | Servings: 4

Ingredients:
- 2 cups frozen green beans
- 5 teaspoons unsalted butter
- 2 teaspoons mustard
- 1/2 teaspoon black pepper
- 1 teaspoon Worcestershire sauce
- 1 tablespoon graham crackers crumbs

Directions:
- Prepare green beans as directed on the package.
- Make a sauce by mixing 2 teaspoons melted butter, mustard, and pepper, and Worcestershire sauce. Heat in the microwave for 30 seconds.
- Toss sauce with hot cooked green beans.
- Mix remaining butter (melted with graham crackers crumbs. Sprinkle on top of the beans and serve.

Nutrition:

• Calories 75, Total Fat 5.4g, Saturated Fat 0.8g, Cholesterol 0mg, Sodium 84mg, Total Carbohydrate 6.1g, Dietary Fiber 2.3g, Total Sugars 1.4g, Protein 1.6g, Calcium 32mg, Iron 1mg, Potassium 132mg, Phosphorus 80 mg

Lemon Green Beans with Almonds

• Preparation Time: 15 minutes | Cooking Time: 15 minutes | Servings: 4 Ingredients:
  • 1/2 cup chopped almonds
  • 1 pound green beans, trimmed and cut into 2 inch pieces
  • 2 1/2 tablespoons olive oil
  • 1 lemon, juiced and zest
  • Salt and pepper to taste

Directions:

   • Preheat the oven to 375 degrees F. Arrange nuts in a single layer on a baking sheet. Toast in the preheated oven until lightly browned, approximately 5 to 10 minutes.

   • Place green beans in a steamer over 1 inch of boiling water, and cover. Steam for 8 to 10 minutes, or until tender, but still bright green.

• Place cooked beans in a large bowl, and toss with olive oil, lemon juice, and lemon zest. Season with salt and pepper. Transfer beans to a serving dish, and sprinkle with toasted almonds. Serve immediately.

Nutrition:

• Calories 211, Total Fat 18.2g, Saturated Fat 1.8g, Cholesterol 0mg, Sodium 7mg, Total Carbohydrate 11g, Dietary Fiber 5.3g, Total Sugars 2.1g, Protein 6g, Calcium 55mg, Iron 2mg, Potassium 339mg, Phosphorus 180 mg

Eggplant Casserole

- Preparation Time: 15 minutes | Cooking Time: 20 minutes | Servings: 4

Ingredients:
- 3 cups eggplant
- 3 large eggs
- 1/8 teaspoon salt
- ½ teaspoon pepper
- ¼ teaspoon sage
- ½ cup white bread crumbs
- 1 tablespoon olive oil

Directions:
- Preheat the oven to 350 degrees F.
- Peel and cut up eggplant. Place eggplant pieces in a pan, cover with water, and boil until tender. Drain and mash.
- Combine beaten eggs, salt, pepper, and sage with mashed eggplant. Place in a greased casserole dish.
- Mix olive oil with white bread crumbs.
- Top the casserole with breadcrumbs and bake for 20 minutes or until the top begins to brown.

Nutrition:

• Calories 153, Total Fat 8.1g, Saturated Fat 1.8g, Cholesterol 140mg, Sodium 226mg, Total Carbohydrate 13.8g, Dietary Fiber 2.9g, Total Sugars 3g, Protein 7.2g, Calcium 52mg, Iron 2mg, Potassium 221mg, Phosphorus 115mg

Garlic Green Beans

- Preparation Time: 10 minutes | Cooking Time: 15 minutes | Servings: 4

Ingredients:
- 1 tablespoon butter
- 3 tablespoons olive oil
- 1 medium head garlic - peeled and sliced
- 2 (14.5 ounces) cans green beans, drained
- Salt and pepper to taste
- ¼ cup grated Parmesan cheese
- 1 teaspoon dried basil

Directions:
- In a large skillet over medium heat, melt butter with olive oil; add garlic, and cook until lightly browned, stirring frequently. Stir in green beans, and season with salt and pepper. Cook until beans are tender, about 10 minutes. Remove from heat, and sprinkle with Parmesan cheese and basil.

Nutrition:

• Calories 96, Total Fat 9.2g, Saturated Fat 2.4g, Cholesterol 6mg, Sodium 27mg, Total Carbohydrate 3.6g, Dietary Fiber 1.3g, Total Sugars 0.5g, Protein 1.3g, Calcium 30mg, Iron 0mg, Potassium 89mg, Phosphorus 71mg

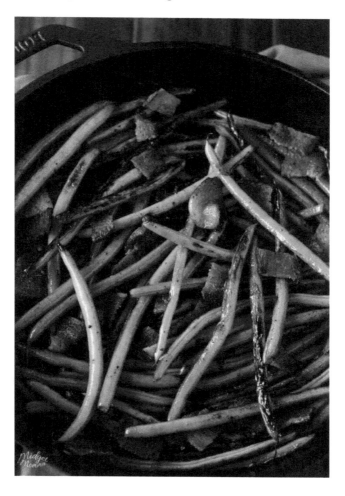

Ginger Veggie Stir-Fry

• Preparation Time: 10 minutes | Cooking Time: 15 minutes | Servings: 4

Ingredients:

- 1 tablespoon corn-starch
- 1 1/2 cloves garlic, crushed
- 2 teaspoons chopped fresh ginger root, divided
- 1/4 cup olive oil, divided
- 1 small head broccoli, cut into florets
- 3/4 cup julienned carrots
- 1/2 cup halved green beans
- ½ tablespoon soy sauce
- 2 1/2 tablespoons water
- 1/4 cup chopped onion

Directions:

• In a large bowl, blend corn-starch, garlic, 1 teaspoon ginger, and 2 tablespoons olive oil until corn-starch is dissolved. Mix in broccoli, carrots, and green beans, tossing to lightly coat.

• Heat the remaining 2 tablespoons oil in a large skillet or wok over medium heat. Cook vegetables in oil for 2 minutes, stirring constantly to prevent burning. Stir in soy sauce and water. Mix in onion and remaining 1 teaspoon ginger. Cook until vegetables are tender but still crisp.

Nutrition:

> • Calories 102, Total Fat 8.5g, Saturated Fat 1.2g, Cholesterol 0mg, Sodium 91mg, Total Carbohydrate 6.5g, Dietary Fiber 1.6g, Total Sugars 1.9g, Protein 1.4g, Calcium 25mg, Iron 1mg, Potassium 154mg, Phosphorus 101mg

Roasted Green Beans

- Preparation Time: 10 minutes | Cooking Time: 25 minutes | Servings: 4

Ingredients:

- 2 pounds fresh green beans, trimmed
- 1 tablespoon olive oil, or as needed
- Salt to taste
- 1/2 teaspoon freshly ground black pepper

Directions:

- Preheat the oven to 400 degrees F.
- Pat green beans dry with paper towels if necessary; spread onto a jelly roll pan. Drizzle with

olive oil and sprinkle with salt and pepper. Use your fingers to coat beans evenly with olive oil and spread them out so they don't overlap.

- Roast in the preheated oven until beans are slightly shriveled and have brown spots, 20 to 25 minutes.

Nutrition:

- Calories 48, Total Fat 3.6g, Saturated Fat

0.5g, Cholesterol 0mg, Sodium 585mg, Total Carbohydrate 4.1g, Dietary Fiber 1.9g, Total Sugars 0.8g, Protein 1g, Calcium 22mg, Iron 1mg, Potassium 118mg, Phosphorus 91mg

French Fries Made with Zucchini

• Preparation Time: 10 minutes | Cooking Time: 25 minutes | Servings: 4

Ingredients:
- 2 medium zucchini
- 1 cup of soy milk
- 2 large eggs
- 3/4 cup corn-starch
- 3/4 cup dry unseasoned bread crumbs
- 3 teaspoons dried basil
- ½ cup olive oil

Directions:

• Peel and slice zucchini into 3/4-inch sticks, 4-inch long. Rinse zucchini and pat dry. • In a medium bowl, mix milk and eggs until well blended. In a wide, shallow bowl, combine

corn-starch, bread crumbs, and basil.
• Heat oil in a frying pan on high heat.
• Dip zucchini sticks into the egg mixture

and then roll each piece in bread crumb mixture. • Place in oil, flipping regularly, and fry for 3 minutes or until golden brown. • Drain on paper towels and serve immediately.

Nutrition:

• Calories 129, Total Fat 11.7g, Saturated Fat 1.8g, Cholesterol 37mg, Sodium 44mg, Total Carbohydrate 4.6g, Dietary Fiber 0.5g, Total Sugars 1.6g, Protein 2.6g, Calcium 19mg, Iron 1mg, Potassium 109mg, Phosphorus 80mg

Garlicky Ginger Eggplant

- Preparation Time: 10 minutes | Cooking Time: 00 minutes | Servings: 4

Ingredients:
- 2 cups eggplant
- 2 teaspoons minced ginger
- 2 garlic cloves
- 1/4 cup fresh Parsley
- 2 tablespoons olive oil
- 1/2 cup fresh mushroom pieces
- 1/4 teaspoon red chili pepper flakes

Directions:

- Slice eggplant into 1-1/2-inch long pieces. Mince garlic cloves. Chop parsley. • Heat olive oil in a large skillet. Add eggplant, ginger, garlic, and mushrooms. Stir-fry over

medium-high heat until eggplant begins to soften, 4-6 minutes.

- Add parsley, chili pepper flakes to eggplant. Continue cooking for 1-2

minutes. Remove
from heat and serve.

Nutrition:

• Calories 78, Total Fat 7.2g, Saturated Fat
1g, Cholesterol 0mg, Sodium 2mg, Total
Carbohydrate 3.9g, Dietary Fiber 1.7g,
Total Sugars 1.4g, Protein 0.9g, Calcium
10mg, Iron 1mg, Potassium 145mg,
Phosphorus 48mg

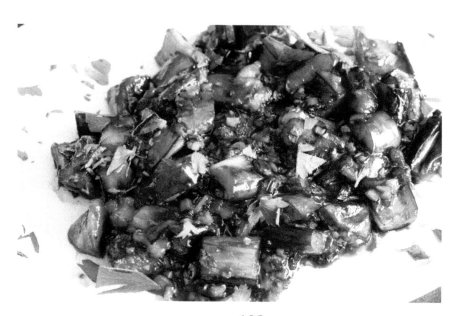

Garlic Kale Buckwheat

- Preparation Time: 10 minutes | Cooking Time: 25 minutes | Servings: 4

Ingredients:

- 2/3 cup water
- 1/3 cup buckwheat
- 1 tablespoon olive oil
- 1 cup chopped kale
- 1 clove garlic, minced
- Salt and ground black pepper to taste

Directions:

- Bring 2/3 cup water and buckwheat to a boil in a saucepan. Reduce heat to medium-low, cover, and simmer until buckwheat is tender and water has been absorbed, 15 to 20 minutes.
- Heat olive oil in a skillet over medium heat; sauté kale and garlic in the hot oil until kale is wilted, about 5 minutes. Season with salt and pepper.
- Stir buckwheat into kale mixture; cook

until flavors blend, about 5 more minutes. Add 1 tablespoon of water to the mixture to keep it from sticking.

Nutrition:

- Calories 88, Total Fat 4g, Saturated Fat 0.6g, Cholesterol 0mg, Sodium 9mg, Total Carbohydrate 12.1g, Dietary Fiber 1.7g, Total Sugars 0g, Protein 2.4g, Calcium 28mg, Iron 1mg, Potassium 151mg, Phosphorus 104mg

Glazed Zucchini

- Preparation Time: 05 minutes | Cooking Time: 10 minutes | Servings: 4

Ingredients:

- 2 cups Zucchini
- 1 tablespoon honey
- 1 teaspoon corn-starch
- 1/8 teaspoon salt
- 1/4 teaspoon ground ginger
- 1/4 cup apple juice
- 2 tablespoons unsalted butter

Directions:

- Slice zucchini into -inch thick slices. Place zucchinis and 1/4 cup water in a pot. Cover and cook until slightly tender.
- Mix honey, corn-starch, salt, ginger, apple juice, and melted butter. Pour mixture over zucchini and water.
- Cook, stirring occasionally, for 10 minutes or until mixture thickens.

Nutrition:

• Calories 86, Total Fat 5.9g, Saturated Fat 3.7g, Cholesterol 15mg, Sodium 121mg, Total Carbohydrate 8.8g, Dietary Fiber 0.7g, Total Sugars 6.8g, Protein 0.8g, Calcium 12mg, Iron 0mg, Potassium 170mg, Phosphorus 56 Mg

Grilled Summer Squash

• Preparation Time: 05 minutes | Cooking Time: 10 minutes | Servings: 4

Ingredients:

- • 2 medium summer squash
- • Non-stick cooking spray
- • 1/4 teaspoon garlic powder
- • 1/4 teaspoon black pepper

Directions:

• Wash summer squash with mild soap and water; rinse well.

• Cut each squash into four pieces; cut both vertically and horizontally.

• Place on a cookie sheet or large platter and spray with non-stick cooking spray. • Sprinkle with garlic powder and black pepper, to taste (both optional).

• Cook on either a gas grill. Cook for approximately three to five minutes, flipping once. The

squash should be tender but not mushy. If cooking on a gas grill, place the flat surface down on a sheet

of aluminum foil sprayed with non-stick cooking
spray.

• Cook approximately 5 to 7 minutes over a
medium flame, watching carefully. Flip and cook
forapproximately 2 more minutes on the ―round‖
side.

Nutrition:

• Calories 17, Total Fat 0.2g, Saturated Fat
0.1g, Cholesterol 0mg, Sodium 2mg, Total
Carbohydrate 3.4g, Dietary Fiber 0.9g,
Total Sugars 3g, Protein 0.9g, Calcium
18mg, Iron 0mg, Potassium 190mg,
Phosphorus100mg

Pineapple and Pepper Curry

- Preparation Time: 05 minutes | Cooking Time: 15 minutes | Servings: 4

Ingredients:
- 2 cups green bell pepper
- 1/2 cup red onion
- 1 tablespoon cilantro
- 1 tablespoon ginger root
- 2 tablespoons olive oil
- 1/2 cup pineapple juice
- 1 teaspoon curry powder
- 1/2 tablespoon lemon juice

Directions:
- Chop bell pepper, onion, and cilantro. Shred ginger root.
- Heat oil and when hot add ginger and red onion. Cook until the onion is transparent. • Microwave peppers on high for 6 minutes. Add the peppers to the onion mixture. Close the

lid of the pan and cook on low for 10 minutes, stirring to avoid burning peppers.

• Add pineapple juice and simmer for 2 minutes. Add curry powder and cilantro. Turn the
 vegetables once and let simmer on low for 2 minutes.

• Garnish lemon juice before serving.

Nutrition:

• Calories 107, Total Fat 6g, Saturated Fat 0.8g, Cholesterol 0mg, Sodium 4mg, Total Carbohydrate 12.5g, Dietary Fiber 2.6g, Total Sugars 7.1g, Protein 2.3g, Calcium 20mg, Iron 1mg, Potassium 222mg, Phosphorus150mg

Lightning Source UK Ltd.
Milton Keynes UK
UKHW020746250621
386136UK00005B/52